PRAISE FOR *THE POCKET GUIDE OF FH FOR NURSES*

As an RN with limited clinical experience in Cardiology, I found this pocket guide very informative on a topic I have very little knowledge about. It is concise and provides all the essential and relevant information pertaining to FH in a portable format that can be readily available to the Clinician working at the bedside.

This pocket guide certainly heightens the bedside Clinicians' awareness of FH, by bringing it to the forefront of the Clinician's mind. It covers everything with its historical recount of FH, the genetics, right through to the diagnosis, management and treatment of FH, including the role the Nurse can play in identifying the undiagnosed FH patient.

A collection of colour images demonstrates signs and symptoms to look out for, as well as an easy to use tool for detection of FH, which is designed to be utilised on a daily basis, thus empowering the bedside Clinician to identify those patients who may present with unrecognised FH.

A great little pocket guide!

Judith Bruechert,
RN, PG CertCritical Care

34. तुमसे दिल की बातें करना

तुमसे दिल की बातें करना
और रातों को तारे गिनना

कभी कभी अच्छा लगता है
कुछ खास पुराने गाने सुनना

तुम कहती हो डर लगता है
हाथ पकड़ कर आगे चलना

आगे मुश्किल भी आएंगी
सोच समझ कर राहें चुनना

सीख लिया है तुमने कैसे
सच्चे झूठे वादे करना

सुन्दर हैं ये गहरी आंखें
इनमें काजल डाले रखना l

www.ingramcontent.com/pod-product-compliance
Lightning Source LLC
Chambersburg PA
CBHW070651240926
51846CB00003BA/868
9789375276906

32. दर्द सहने के लिये मजबूर हो जायेंगे

दर्द सहने के लिये मजबूर हो जायेंगे
मत कुरेदो ये ज़ख्म नासूर हो जाएंगे

खिला रहे हो जिनको अपनी चोंच का दाना
ऐसे उड़ेंगे एक दिन बहुत दूर हो जायेंगे

इठला रहे हैं आज जो अपनी चमक पे
फूल मुरझाने के बाद बेनूर हो जायेंगे

मुझ पर ही इल्ज़ाम आयेगा इस बेवफ़ाई का
वो मेरी जान लेकर भी बेकसूर हो जायेंगे

लिखने वालों को चाहे भुला दे जमाना
किरदार कहानी के मग़र मशहूर हो जायेंगे I

33. ये दर्दे दिल है जो आँखों से निकल रहा है

ये दर्दे दिल है जो आँखों से निकल रहा है
वो मौसम तो नहीं फिर कैसे बदल रहा है

मेरी आँखों के आगे आज ये मंजर है कैसा
ना जाने कौन उसका हाथ थामे चल रहा है

मैं अपने आप को दुश्मन से तो महफ़ूज़ कर लूँ
मगर ये कौन है जो दोस्त बनके छल रहा है

हकीक़त से नहीं इसका कोई भी वास्ता है
ये झूठा ख़्वाब है पलकों के नीचे पल रहा है

चलो अच्छा है सर्दी में तुम अपने हाथ सेकों
मैं जाके देखता हूँ मेरा घर कैसे जल रहा है I

A Pocket Guide of FH for NURSES

Detection and Diagnosis of Familial HYPERCHOLESTROLAEMIA

FIRST EDITION

Jackie Ryan NP, MNurs(NURSPract),
MNurs, GDipHlthSc, Cert(CC).
Adjunct Research Fellow, University
of Western Australia

Laurie Kear, RN, MHlthSc(CDM),
GCert(HlthMgt), CCRC.
Adjunct Research Fellow,
Griffith University, Queensland

A Pocket Guide of FH for Nurses

Detection and Diagnosis of Familial Hypercholestrolaemia

First Edition - 2023 - v3.03 - 190224

This book is intended as a reference guide for nurses. It is not a medical manual, nor is it intended as a substitute for any health intervention that may be prescribed by a medical practitioner for the treatment of Familial Hypercholestrolaemia (FH).

Internet addresses and hyperlinks cited in this book were accurate when it went to press.

Book Layout www.EvolveGlobalPublishing.com

ASIN: B0CQDY8NFJ (Amazon Kindle)
ISBN: 978-0-6486270-2-9 (eBook)
ISBN: 978-0-6486270-0-5 (Amazon Paperback)
ISBN: 978-0-6486270-1-2 (Amazon Hardcover)
ISBN: 978-0-6486270-4-3 (Ingram Spark) PAPERBACK
ISBN: 978-0-6486270-5-0 (Ingram Spark) HARDCOVER
ISBN: 978-0-6486270-3-6 (Smashwords)

Figure 1 - reproduced with permission of Professor Joseph L Goldstein
Pictures A and B - reproduced with permission from Dr Warrick Bishop
Picture C - reproduced with permission from Prefessor Gerald Watts
Other images subject to unrestricted use under creative commons 2.5.

ABOUT THE AUTHORS

Jackie Ryan has a varied nursing background incorporating many years in Coronary Care. She is a Nurse Practitioner specialising in Cardiometabolic Disorder Assessment and Diagnostic Services, she operates her private practice *'Perth Lipid Clinic'* from a general practice in addition to her practice at the Cardiovascular Services rooms at Hollywood Private Hospital.

As a Nurse Practitioner (NP), Jackie specialises in the diagnosis, treatment and management of cardiometabolic disorders, in particular Familial Hypercholestrolaemia, employing cascade screening to diagnose and then treat a wider range of patients affected. Jackie is an Adjunct Research Fellow with the School of Medicine and Pharmacology at the University of Western Australia.

Laurie Kear is clinical research professional and registered nurse with a diverse background in the clinical and operational management of research programs. She has worked in public and private health services and academic research organizations across Australia.

Her clinical research experience has involved hundreds of clinical trials across a broad range of therapeutic areas and trial phases, including early phase trials of new medicines for the treatment of Familial Hypercholestrolaemia. Laurie is an Adjunct Senior Clinical Research Fellow with the Institute of Glycomics at Griffith University's Queensland Gold Coast Campus.

FOREWORD

Familial hypercholesterolemia has an enormous impact on individuals, loved ones, family, friends, the community, and the healthcare dollar.

A problem exists. Collectively, as a medical community, we are failing at early identification of and early intervention for this common, inherited condition. An urgency surrounds it. With timely identification and proper treatment, community pain, loss, morbidity, and mortality could be minimised.

Despite these issues, champions in the field exist. Individuals are making a career from a passion for saving lives through appropriate care and identifying individuals at high risk well before sufferers realise there could be a problem.

Jackie Ryan is one of those Giants.

Unquestionably, she is a leading nurse practitioner in this space in Australia, being highly regarded at home and overseas.

"A Pocket Guide of FH for Nurses" is a wonderful resource. This little treasure pulls together Jackie's years of experience and up-to-date information on the genetics and treatment of familial hypercholesterolemia.

Most importantly, however, it highlights how nurses at the coal face of care can initiate steps to make real and meaningful differences in people's lives.

I know this book will live in the pockets of nurses in coronary care units, cardiology wards, general practice settings, and, of course, lipid clinics, as a practical resource to help support the delivery of the best care.

Dr Warrick Bishop MBBS, FRACP
cardiologist
best-selling author
change maker and educator
helping people live as well as possible for as long as possible

TABLE OF CONTENTS

INTRODUCTION

During the 1970's, whilst working as a Registered Nurse in the Coronary Care Unit at the Royal Prince Alfred Hospital in Sydney, I observed at least once or twice a year, seemingly fit, young men and women being admitted to the Coronary Care Unit after suffering an acute cardiac event and I recall that suddenly, sometimes they died!

At the time, my colleagues and I often asked ourselves why did this happen to someone so young and was there anything we as nurses could have done to alter their outcome?

Now, fifty years onwards, we know so much more about the role genetics plays in determining the inheritance of disorders or diseases. Familial Hypercholesterolaemia (FH) is one such disorder. It is present from birth and is characterised by markedly elevated "bad cholesterol" or low-density lipoprotein concentrations and, if left untreated, can lead to premature atherosclerosis, coronary artery disease and death.

Now as a Cardiometabolic Nurse Practitioner, with a keen interest in FH, I specialise in lifestyle advice, diagnostic investigations, cholesterol management and cascade screening, where necessary, for patients with elevated cholesterol levels.

Through a process of clinical assessment and screening, a patient proven to have phenotypic FH, can be referred for genetic testing unless they elect not to have the test.

As nurses we can play a pivotal role in the identification of patients who have FH.

This book is specifically intended to be a guide for nurses to help them in identifying patients, using the FH tools described in this book.

An additional aim of this guide is to assist nurses in the education of patients and their families regarding the benefits of early detection and treatment of hypercholesterolaemia in order to prevent premature heart attack and stroke.

CHAPTER 1

WHAT IS FAMILIAL HYPERCHOLESTEROLAEMIA

History of Identification

First reports of FH were described in the literature toward the end of the 18th century. Then between 1925 and 1938, a Norwegian pathologist named Francis Harbitz's (1867-1950), reported on several cases of sudden death and xanthomatosis.

Xanthomatosis is described as an accumulation of excess lipids in the body due to disturbance of lipid metabolism, marked by the formation of foam cells in skin lesions, called xanthomas. Harbitz noted that there were microscopic peculiarities of the xanthomatosis, more specifically in the characteristics of the foam cells. Foam cells play a central role in the pathogenesis of Atherosclerosis (AS).

Carl Müller (1886-1983) between 1936 and 1938 continued pursuing Harbitz's concepts and studied 17 families with known heart disease in Oslo. In 1938, he published his findings describing a familial pattern of xanthomatosis, hypercholesterolaemia and coronary heart disease[1].

In the families he studied, Müller found xanthomatosis and hypercholesterolaemia were common and that there was a dominate trait amongst family members. He suggested the occurrence of heart disease in families should alert clinicians to suspect the possibility of a disorder he called familial hypercholesterolaemia and that prophylactic treatment might by pertinent for patients who show signs of FH. For more than 50 years his suggestion of prophylactic treatment was not followed by clinicians.

Dr. Avedis Khachadurian (1926-2022) through his research into families in Lebanon during the 1960s and 1970s[2,3,] showed that children with signs of hypercholesterolemia had inherited two aberrant genes leading to overproduction of cholesterol and premature death from coronary artery disease. These important observations defined the disorder known as homozygous familial hypercholesterolemia (HoFH).

Later two doctors based at the University of Texas USA, Michael S. Brown and Joseph L. Goldstein, published important findings[4, 5, 6, 7] about the regulation of cholesterol metabolism and the treatment of diseases caused by abnormally elevated cholesterol levels in the blood.

Brown and Goldstein's research into cholesterol metabolism and more specifically the LDL-C receptor[8] won them the

Noble Prize for Medicine in 1985. This discovery forms the foundation for our present knowledge concerning cholesterol metabolism and has led to new principles for treatment and prevention of atherosclerosis.

Leiv Ose in 2008[9] highlighted in his publication "The Real Code of Leonardo da Vinci" that nearly 500 years before the research of Harbitz, Müller, Brown and Goldstein, the famous Italian artist and scientist Leonardo Da Vinci in his painting of Madonna Lisa Maria de Gherardini (Mona Lisa) depicted pictorial evidence of the clinical signs of FH. This painting is thought to be the earliest documentation of FH.

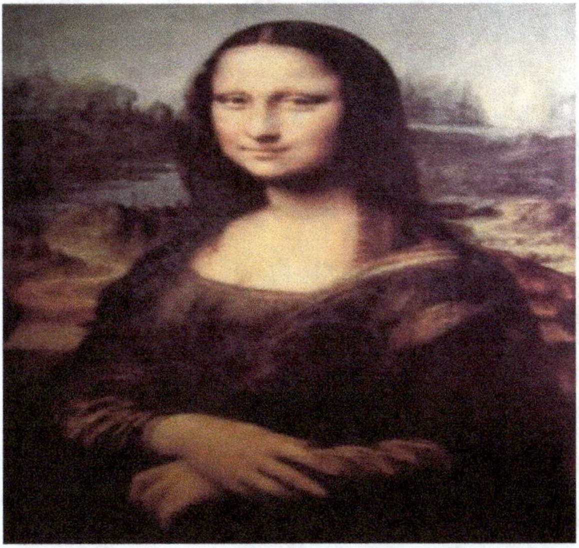

©2008 Bentham Science Publishers Ltd CC BY-SA 2.5 DEED

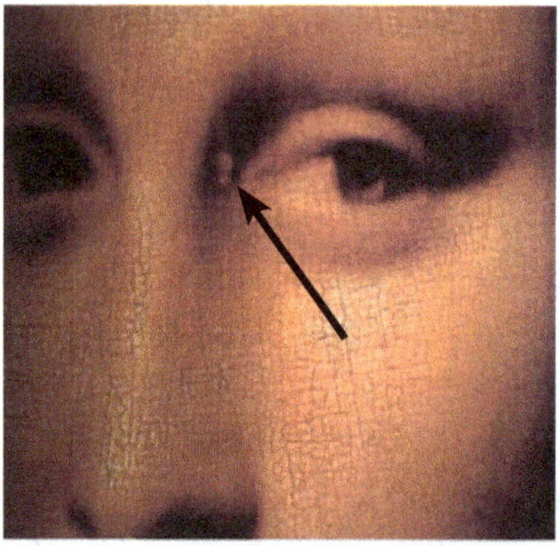

A closer review of her eye area reveals: "a yellow irregular leather-like spot at the inner end of the left upper eyelid"[9]

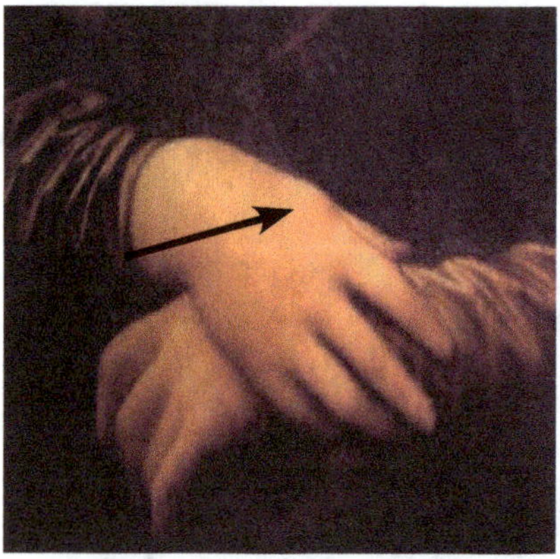

"A soft bumpy well-defined swelling is revealed on the dorsum of the right hand beneath the index finger being about 3cm long"[9]

The Basic Science

In their early scientific research, Brown and Goldstein[5] cultured cells (fibroblasts) from healthy people and those with FH. Cultured fibroblasts cells need cholesterol (in the form of LDL) in their cell membranes. They found that LDL was taken up by highly specific receptor molecules (LDL-receptors) that sit on the cell surface. They then made a revolutionary discovery that fibroblasts from patients with the most severe form of FH - homozygous FH (HoFH) completely lacked functional LDL-receptors and the fibroblasts from patients with the milder form of FH - heterozygous FH (HeFH) had fewer LDL-receptors than normal.

In later studies Brown and Goldstein[7, 8] showed that LDL, which had bound to the receptor, was taken up by the cells as an LDL-receptor complex. The receptor is localised on the cell surface in what is called a coated pit or vesicle (Figure 1).

The cholesterol in the LDL particle is released inside the liver. One effect of the uptake of cholesterol is that it inhibits the manufacture of new LDL-receptors on the surface of the cell. Therefore, a reduced number of LDL-receptors lead to a diminished LDL uptake by the liver resulting in increased levels of circulating LDL in the blood. Hence there is a risk of accumulation in the arterial walls.

Figure 1

Sequential steps in the LDL receptor pathway of mammalian cells (modified by Brown and Goldstein)[10].

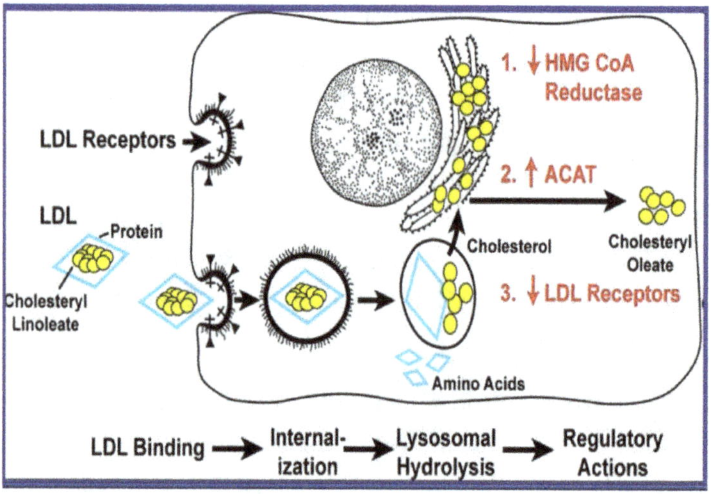

(Reproduced with permission of Professor Joseph L. Goldstein)

This important discovery of the LDL-C receptor is what led to them being awarded the Nobel Prize in 1985.

CHAPTER 2

THE GENETICS OF FH

Overview

FH is a common inherited (i.e., genetic) autosomal co-dominant disorder with almost complete penetrance, which is present from birth and characterized by high serum cholesterol levels, specifically very high levels of low-density lipoprotein(LDL), often referred to as "bad cholesterol" in the blood, which can lead specifically to the development of premature atherosclerosis of the proximal segment of the coronary arteries and aorta, and in severe cases supravalvular aortic stenosis. It is one of the most common disorders of lipid metabolism.

People who inherit from a single parent one abnormal copy of, the LDLR, APOB or PCSK9 gene (which affect how a body regulates and removes cholesterol from the blood) could have HeFH. The most common genetic defect is in the LDLR (approximately 90%). Defects in the other two genes are rare. Males with HeFH may develop premature CVD as early as 30 to 40 years of age, women approximately a decade later.

If a person inherits an abnormal gene from both of their parents, then they will have HoFH, which leads to a more severe form of the disease in childhood that will require early intervention to prevent CVD. All newly identified cases of FH should be offered genetic counselling pre and post genetic testing.

There are other factors such as the genetic founder effect, that can influence the prevalence of FH in populations, or penetrance that determines physical traits that are inherited by an individual.

Founder effect

Founder effect is the loss of genetic variation that occurs when a population is established by a very small number of individuals. This can occur when migrants that are not genetically representative of a population migrate to another geographic area. Inbreeding within a smaller group can result in a higher incidence of FH as increased genetic drift results in a decreased genetic variation[11, 12].

The founder effect is thought to be responsible for the prevalence of FH associated variants amongst Finns, Icelanders, Christian Lebanese, Tunisians, Gujarati South African Indians, Ashkenazi Jews, South African Afrikaners and French Canadians[12].

Penetrance

Penetrance describes how likely a person is to present a specific physical trait based on their genetic profile. Traits are physical features that are coded in a person's DNA. In this case, FH is the trait. The penetrance of FH is >90%, which means if a person's 1st degree relative has FH, then they have a "high likelihood" of inheriting the FH disorder and males and females can be equally affected[13]. Therefore, DNA variations affecting the gene increase the risks of developing FH, but they <u>don't guarantee it</u>. This is known as *incomplete penetrance.*

The burden of LDL-C in an individual is dependent on the type of FH genetic defect they have. Figure 2 depicts the cumulative exposure (i.e., cholesterol year score) by age in those with HeFH, HoFH and in healthy individuals.

Figure 2

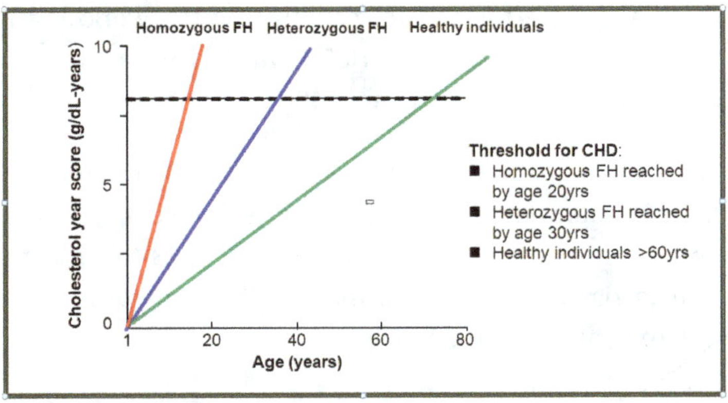

Adapted from Horton et al. J Lipid Res. 2009;50:S172-S177[14]

Prevalence

Worldwide

FH is the most common autosomal-dominant, monogenetic disorder, estimated to affect about 30 million worldwide, and is characterized by lifelong highly elevated low-density lipoprotein (LDL) cholesterol levels and thus an increased risk for ischemic heart disease (IHD)[15].

For years, the prevalence of heterozygous FH in the general population was believed to be 1:500, and the estimated HoFH prevalence 1:1,000,000.

However, a recent meta-analysis by Beheshti et.al, (2020) found that of the 197 countries in the world only 17 (9%) have reported the prevalence of FH in their general populations and an additional 4 countries have reported prevalence in their founder populations[15]. Therefore, the prevalence of FH in 90% of countries in the world is still unknown. The prevalence of HoFH, which is much rarer, has been is estimated to be about 1:400,000.

Their meta-analysis of 104 studies (11 million subjects) from 21 countries found the prevalence of FH in the general population to be 1:313 and that FH is up to 23-fold greater in high risk groups such as those with premature IHD or severe hypercholestrolaemia[15].

The following figure adapted from Beheshti et.al, (2020)[15] illustrates their findings regarding the prevalence of FH in the general populations and in those diagnosed with ischaemic heart disease or severe hypercholestrolaemia.

Figure 3 Prevalence of Familial Hypercholestrolaemia

(Adapted from Beheshti, S.O. et al. J Am Coll Cardiol. 2020;75(20):2553-66)

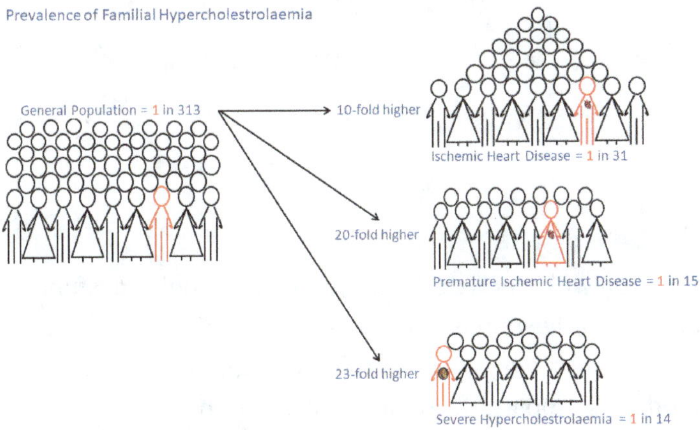

The prevalence of FH is as high as 1:200 in certain founder groups or populations and has been estimated to be as high as 1:67 in the Ashkenazi Jew population in South Africa, who are descendants from the Jewish peoples who emigrated from a small geographical area in Lithuania between 1880 and 1910[16].

FH Prevalence in Australia

(Diagram adapted from the FH Australasia Network site)

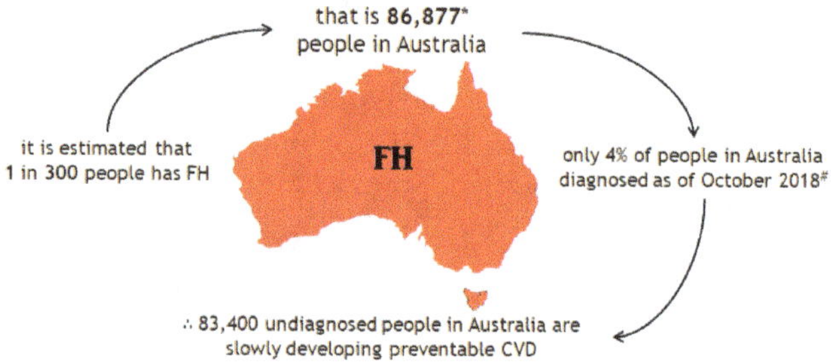

* based on Australian Bureau of Statistics total population figures Population clock (abs.gov.au) as of March 2023

Pang J.; Chen D.C.; et. al. Comparative aspects of the care of familial hypercholesterolemia in the "Ten Countries Study" J. Clin. Lipid. (2019) 13, 287-300[17]

Disease Burden

Children with HeFH develop signs of endothelial dysfunction and the earliest phase of atherosclerosis at an early age and by 10 years of age, significant thickening of the carotid intima-media is apparent. Additionally, coronary angiographic studies in those with HeFH reveal clear evidence of stenotic lesions in approximately 25% of children or young adults between the ages of 11 and 23.

Low-Density Lipoprotein Cholesterol (LDL-C) is a strong and independent predictor of arterial thickening in children with HeFH and the accumulated arterial wall damage during childhood years if left untreated dramatically increases the risk for CAD in HeFH patients after the age of 20 years[17, 18].

An integrated guidance published by Horton et al. (2022) recommends a number of screening and testing strategies for children and adolescence suspected of having HeFH[19].

Morbidity and Mortality

It is estimated that around 50% of untreated FH-affected men experience adverse events by 50 years of age while women with a similar degree of cholesterol elevation experience adverse events approximately a decade later. If left untreated they are at higher risk of dying due to sudden cardiovascular events.

Historical information available from a large eight generation Dutch family traced back to a single pair of ancestors in the 19 century revealed an overall 3.26 fold greater relative risk of mortality among those presumed to have heterozygous FH, although the pedigree also revealed individuals who must have inherited the gene mutation responsible for FH and who lived a normal life span[20].

CHAPTER 3

SCREENING FOR FH

Phenotypic Detection of Proband Cases

Accepted guidelines recommend applying both a systematic and opportunistic approach to screening for FH[19,21,22,23]. An opportunistic approach can be successfully implemented as part of the nurses' or other health professionals normal health assessment.

In both Primary Care and Hospital settings, the most feasible methodology to establishing a diagnosis of FH is by applying a clinical phenotypic approach. Essentially this is an assessment of the level of hypercholesterolaemia, the length of time an individual has been exposed to these high levels and the family history of CVD that determines an individual's cardiovascular risk.

In the hospital setting in areas such as CCU, cardiac rehabilitation, cardiac wards, and cardiac catheterisation units, nurses and other health professionals who conduct initial assessments can play a pivotal role in the early detection of patient with FH. Putting alerts on cholesterol laboratory reports can also assist primary care doctors, private and hospital specialists to identify potential FH proband cases.

Any patient seen with CVD, who is less than 60 years of age and has a high untreated LDL-C concentration, should be considered to possibly have FH and be investigated further.

Research has shown the potential benefits of screening in CCU to identify patients at high risk for FH allowing management to be optimized, both for diagnosis and therapeutic purposes[23].

Screening for FH in CCU and other units affords a unique opportunity for detecting previously undiagnosed individuals. More importantly the identification of a proband case can trigger the 'Cascade Screening' of relatives, allowing earlier intervention and risk reduction of ASCVD in the family members of newly identified FH patients.

Once a possible FH proband case has been identified, either in the primary care setting or in a hospital setting, they need to be referred to a specialist lipid clinic, cardiologist, or endocrinologist for confirmation of their diagnosis.

Cascade Screening

Cascade Screening is a process for identifying blood related family members of a proband case who may possibly have inherited the FH gene. This method of screening is more cost effective than universal screening[23].

Following Confirmation of Diagnosis

Once the phenotypic diagnosis of FH has been confirmed in the proband case the subsequent step is to construct a Pedigree (sometimes referred to as a progeny tree).

A pedigree helps to explain and follow inheritance in a graphic format, and it is used to systematically screen family members who may be at risk for FH. The components of a pedigree are explained in Chapter 5.

When other family members are identified through the pedigree as being at potential risk, then cascade testing of them should be offered with the permission of both the proband case and the family member.

Cascade testing can occur either in a specialist lipid clinic or via the individual's primary care physician, cardiologist, or endocrinologist.

CHAPTER 4

DIAGNOSIS OF FH

In patients with FH, the capacity of the liver to breakdown LDL-C in a controlled manner is impaired. Consequently, the time period that LDL-C resides in plasma is prolonged, and the tendency of cholesterol particles to undergo oxidation is increased. These oxidised particles in the artery wall can lead to formation of cholesterol-laden 'foam cells', the hallmark of atherosclerotic plaque, with subsequent risk of clinical manifestations[25] such as ACS, MI and sudden death.

The primary, phenotypic diagnostic criteria for FH in adults include: an elevated LDL-cholesterol concentration on two separate occasions, a strong personal and/or family history of elevated cholesterol, premature CVD, the presence of tendon xanthomata and/or arcus cornealis before the age of 45 years in a person or their 1st degree relative(s). Xanthoma in young children is highly suggestive of HoFH[26].

In children suspected of having FH a non-fasting lipid profile should be undertaken initially, with a repeat fasting test if FH is still suspected[26].

Gathering information is important to making a diagnosis as FH is a co-dominantly inherited disease and does not skip a generation.

As previously mentioned, it is important to draw a pedigree to show the line of descent of FH in individuals and those family members who are at risk of having FH.

There are physical signs and symptoms of FH in adults. Some are subtle and can easily be missed. A patient however may have none of the clinical signs but still have FH.

Clinical Signs in FH

(Pictures A, B reproduced with permission from Dr Warrick Bishop)

The most specific sign of FH in an adult is the evidence of Xanthomata of the Achilles tendon, however not all patients will develop these. Xanthomata are more common in those with HoFH and never seen in children with HeFH.

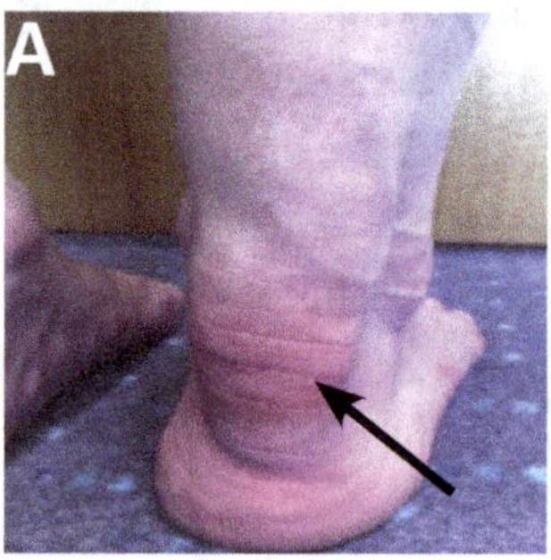

Picture A

Achilles tendon Xanthomata – usually diagnostic of FH

Swollen tendons on the knuckles of the hands like fatty lumps are also a sign of possible FH in adults and may be seen in untreated children with HoFH.

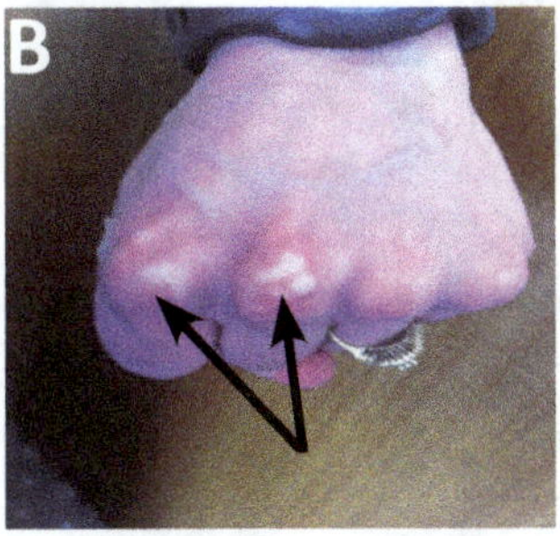

Picture B

Xanthomata on extensor tendons of the hand

A white arc or ring around the edge of the iris of the eye is known as an Arcus cornealis. If seen in individuals younger than 45 years, this may be a sign of possible FH.

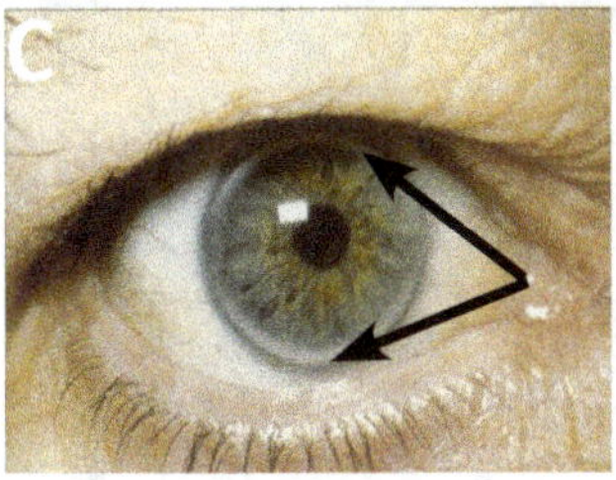

Picture C

Arcus cornealis

(Picture C reproduced with permission from Prof Gerald Watts)

Before a diagnosis of FH can be made it is important to exclude secondary causes of hypercholesterolaemia. The following table adapted from of the Integrated Guidance for Enhancing the Care of Patients with FH in Australia (2021)[32] is a list the lifestyle factors, clinical conditions, and drugs that may increase plasma LDL-C concentration.

It is important to review a patient's diet because increased consumption of low-carbohydrate high-fat diets and ketogenic diets will significantly raise LDL levels, particularly in selected susceptible individuals.

Table 1 Lifestyle factors, clinical conditions and drugs that may increase LDL-C

Adapted from Integrated Guidance for Enhancing the Care of Patients with FH in Australia (2021)

Lifestyle factors
Excess energy intake
High saturated fat diet
High trans-fat diet
Weight gain
Physical inactivity
Clinical conditions
Chronic kidney disease
Nephrotic syndrome
Obstructive liver disease
Human immunodeficiency virus infection
Systemic lupus erythematosus
Hypothyroidism
Pregnancy
Polycystic ovary syndrome
Anorexia nervosa
Menopause
Drugs
Some progestins (norethindrone)
Anabolic steroids
Danazol
Isotretinoin
Immunosuppressives (cyclosporine)
Amiodarone
Thiazide diuretics
Glucocorticoids
Thiazolidinediones (rosiglitazone)
Fibric acids (in severe hypertriglyceridaemia)
Omega-3 fatty acids (in severe hypertriglyceridaemia)

LDL-C Levels

The classic feature of FH is a marked elevation in plasma LDL-C levels from birth. This is due to a genetic defect that impairs the liver's ability to clear LDL-C via the LDL receptor. Extensive research has confirmed that LDL particles play a causal role in the initiation and development of atherosclerotic cardiovascular disease (ASCVD)[29].

As mentioned earlier, patients should have a full fasting cholesterol profile blood test performed on two separate occasions and have elevated LDL-C results. These tests should not be undertaken during periods of illness.

FH should always be considered in adults with a total cholesterol level of ≥7.5mmol/L or an LDL-C level of ≥5.0mmol/L, especially if there is a personal or family history of premature CVD[30].

Lipoprotein (a)

Lipoprotein (a) is a separate genetically inherited disorder. At present it is not well understood, but high levels of Lp(a) are associated with increased risk of CVD.

One in five (1:5) of the general population has elevated Lp(a) and one in three (1:3) individuals who have FH also has elevated Lp(a)[athero.org.au]. Patients with genetically confirmed FH and an elevated Lp(a) are at 10 times greater risk of CAD.

CHAPTER 5

DIAGNOSTIC TOOLS USED IN FH

Diagnostic tools used to establish a phenotypic diagnosis of FH in adults include a combination of cholesterol values, clinical signs, personal and family history of premature CVD.

A universal diagnostic tool has not been established for use in adults. In Australia the Dutch Lipid Clinic Network Score (DLCNS) is used to make a probable or definite clinical diagnosis of FH on the basis of phenotypic criteria[27].

The example of the DLCNS tool on page 27 includes space to draw a pedigree and when used in conjunction with the Cardiovascular Assessment Form (CAF) on page 28 allows a clinician to clearly capture all of the information needed to establish if a possible FH diagnosis is present.

The inpatient admission process within hospitals is an ideal opportunistic screening setting as it involves discussion, assessment, observation and documentation. Through knowledge and awareness of FH nurses can be empowered to be active in the fact-finding process involved in the identification of patients. These tools can be easily incorporated into the routine patient care processes or used when new patients are admitted to hospital.

E:

Lp(a)__________g/L

Lp(a)__________nmol/L

ApoB:__________g/L

CONSENT to Rx ☐

FH REGISTRY: ☐

Patient #

Name:______________________
DOB: ___/___/_____ Age: ____
Address:______________________
____
__________Post Code:______
Mob:______________________
Hm:______________________

GP:

	Dutch Lipid Clinic Network Criteria for FH Diagnosis	Score	Patient Score	Score updates
1.0	**Family History**			
1.1	First degree relatives with known premature coronary and vascular disease (Men < 55 years, Females < 60 years) **Father / Mother / Other:**__________	1		
1.2	**OR** First degree relatives with known LDL-cholesterol (LDL-C) above the 95th percentile (for age and sex) **Father / Mother / Other:**__________			
1.3	First degree relatives with tendinous xanthomata and/or arcus cornealis,	2		
1.4	**OR** Have children aged less than 18 years with LDL-C above the 95th percentile for age and sex			
2.0	**Clinical History**			
2.1	Patient with premature coronary artery disease (Men < 55 years, Females < 60 years)	2		
2.2	Patient with premature cerebral or peripheral vascular disease (Men < 55 years, Females < 60 years)	1		
3.0	**Physical examination**			
3.1	Tendinous xanthomata **Right / Left / Bilateral**	6		
3.2	Arcus cornealis prior to age 45 years **Right / Left / Bilateral**	4		
4.0	**Low Density Lipoprotein Cholesterol, LDL-C (mmol/L)**			
4.1	LDL-C ≥ 8.5	8		
4.2	LDL-C 6.5-8.4	5		
4.3	LDL-C 5.0-6.4	3		
4.4	LDL-C 4.0-4.9	1		
		Phenotypic score:		
5.0	**DNA analysis**			
5.1	Functional mutation in the LDLR, APOB, PCSK9 gene	8		
		Score with DNA testing:		

Family Tree-(Progeny)

TARGET LDL: __________________

FH Diagnostic Categories

Definite	> 8
Probable	6 – 8
Possible	3 – 5
Unlikely	0 – 2

____

Name:

____

Cardiovascular Assessment Form (CAF)

Adapted with permission from a CAF developed by FHWA Nursing Team, RPH (2008).

DATE OF INITIAL ASSESSMENT: / / **PATIENT ID #:** **Name:**

Ht: ______cm **Wt:** ______kg **BMI:** ______kg/m² **Waist** ______cm

(L) BP/HR: 1.______/___ mmHg HR: ___ 2.______/___ mmHg HR: ___ 3.______/___ mmHg HR: ___

(R) BP/HR: 1.______/___ mmHg HR: ___ 2.______/___ mmHg HR: ___ 3.______/___ mmHg HR: ___

Smoking Hx: Never ☐ Former ☐ Current ☐ #/day: _____ Start Age: ____ Stop Age: _____

Alcohol Hx: Never ☐ Rare ☐ Daily ☐ #AFD/wk: ____ Units/week: ____ **Exercise:** Yes No: ☐ Mostly ☐

Diet Heart Healthy: Yes ☐ No: ☐ Mostly ☐ **Low salt:** Yes ☐ No: ☐ Mostly ***Other Diet:***______________

Cardiovascular Hx :

		Age at onset		*Age at onset*
	Hypertension	________	Hypothyroidism	________
	Diabetes	________	Peripheral numbness / tingling	________
	Intermittent claudication	________	Depression or anxiety	________
			Age Onset of Menopause	________
Previous	Angina	________	TIA	________
	MI	________	CVA	________
	Angioplasty / stent	________	Aortic aneurysm repair	________
	CABG	________	Carotid endarterectomy	________
	Fem Bypass Graft	________	Obstructive Sleep Apnoea:	Yes ☐ No: ☐
			Neck Circumference: _____cm **CPAP**:	Yes ☐ No: ☐

CCS: Yes ☐ No: ☐ CCS: _____ *Date:*________ **CTCA**: Yes ☐ No: ☐ *Date:*________ *Summary:* ______________

A'Gram: Yes ☐ No: ☐ *Date:*________ **EST**: Yes ☐ No: ☐ *Date:*________ **Echocardiogram**: Yes ☐ No: ☐ *Date:*_______

Other____

Ethnic Origin:______________________ **Occupation:**______________________

Drug Allergies:

Current Medication				Blood Results	Date					
Name	Dose	Freq.	Start Date	Test						
				TC						
				TG						
				HDL						
				LDL						
				ApoB						
				Lp(a)						
				CK						
				ALT						
				Glucose						
				HbA1c						
				Urea						
				Creat						
				Hb						
				Platelets						
				TSH						

The CAF provides a comprehensive initial overview of the patient's cardiovascular history on admission and the DLCNS allows a risk score to be determined and an early pedigree to be constructed. These tools keep the information gathered succinct and in the one place and can be an excellent reference for later comparisons.

Drawing a Pedigree

A pedigree drawn in a graphic format is used in FH to identify family members who may be at risk.

When drawing a pedigree you start the process with the proband case (which is usually the index case) that has been identified as having the genetic condition FH, or who is concerned that they are at risk of having FH.

The first person in a family who brings the concern of this genetic disorder to the attention of healthcare professionals is usually the index case however; there may be several index cases within an extended family group depending on the cycles of cascade testing undertaken.

Pedigree Symbols

Symbol	Name	Description
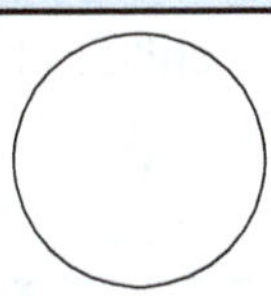	Female	A pedigree symbol circle represents an individual whose gender is female. Individuals are the main component of a pedigree chart.

	Male	A pedigree symbol square represents an individual whose gender is male.
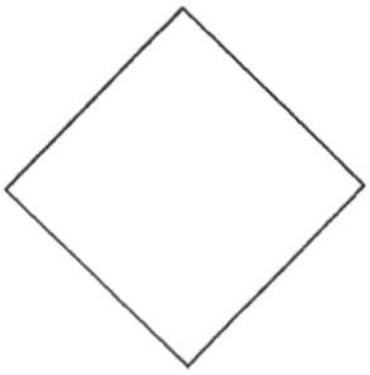	Unknown Gender	An individual of unknown or undetermined gender.
	Positive Female	A female who is affected by the disease.
	Positive Male	A male individual who is affected by the disease.
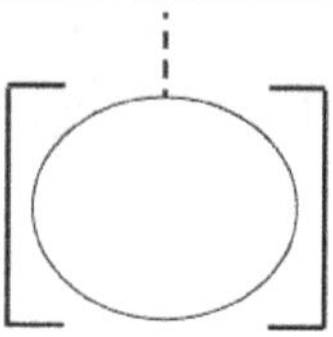	Adopted Female	Adopted female child in the family.
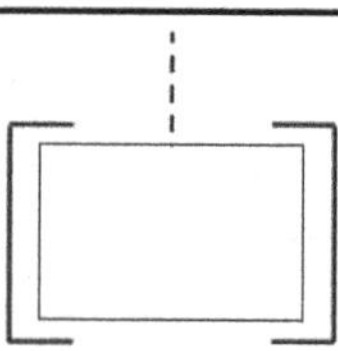	Adopted Male	Adopted male child in the family.

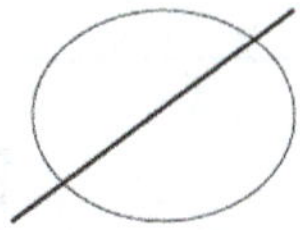	Deceased Female	Deceased female. The age of the member at death will go under the symbol.
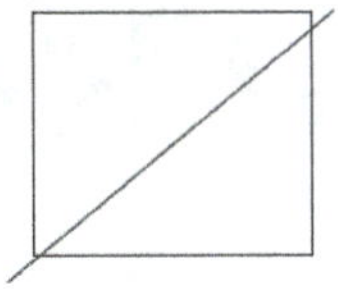	Deceased Male	Deceased male individual. The age of the member at death will go under the symbol.

Pedigree Relationship Lines

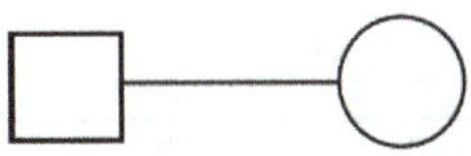	Are horizontal lines that show marriage, divorce, or another relationship status. A horizontal line runs parallel to the x-axis.
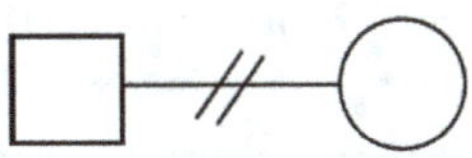	

Line of Decent

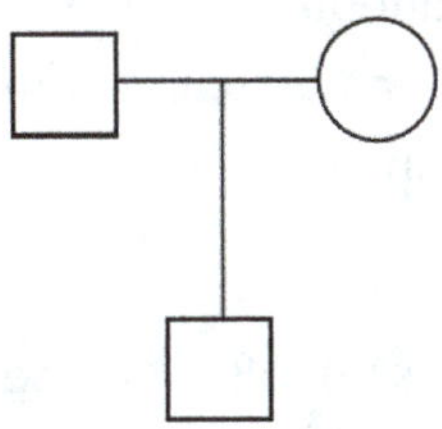	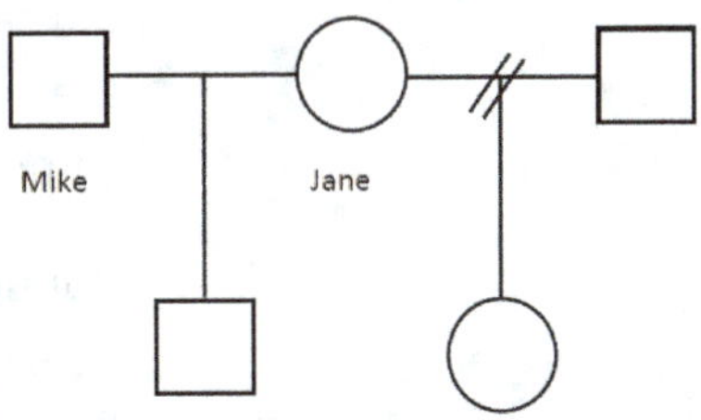
A vertical relationship line is a line of descent that shows the relationship and transmission of traits or diseases from the previous generation. A break or disjoint shows a broken relationship.	

Sibling Lines

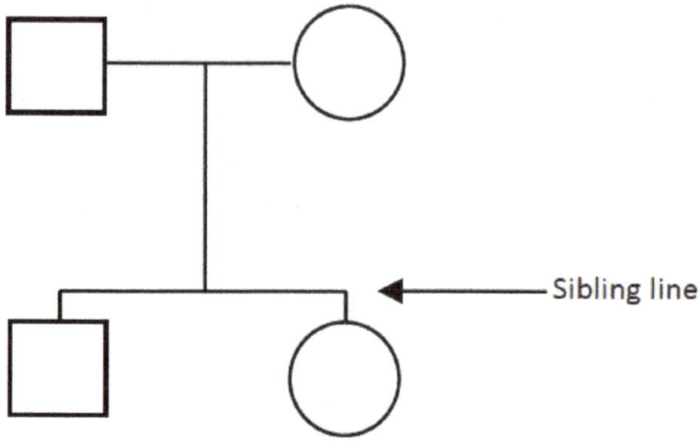

The siblings are connected through a horizontal sibling pedigree symbol. The siblings are placed in order of birth from left to right.

Consanguinity symbols

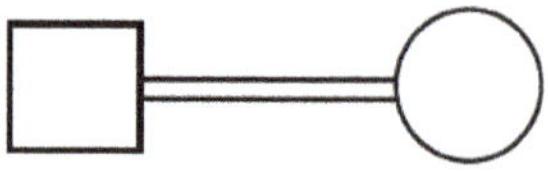

Consanguineous matings are when individuals share a common ancestor.

Double lines between pedigree symbols represent it. If the degree of relationship is not obvious from pedigree hierarchy, it is stated above the relationship line.
e.g., third cousins

Multiple Birth symbols

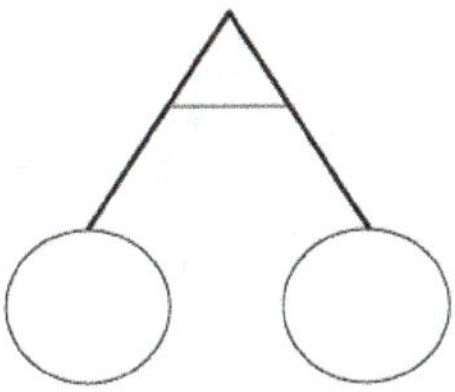	Monozygotic twins are identical twins represented by horizontal lines connecting the two diagonal lines that lead down to the gender symbols.
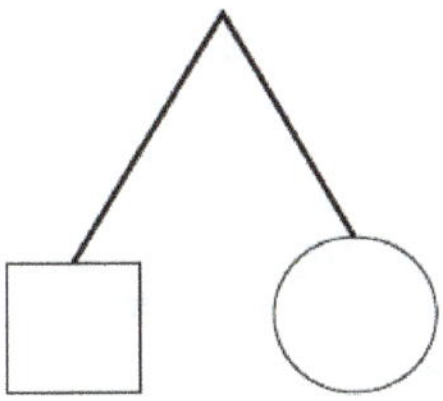	Dizygotic Twins are non-identical twins. They are represented by two diagonal, vertical lines coming from the same point of origin. This is an example of brother and sister dizygotic twins.

No children symbols

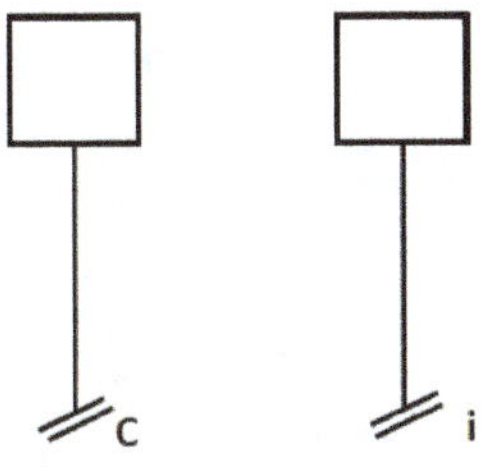	No children of a member are represented by a vertical line with two hash marks at the end. A 'c' letter Indicates that an adult does not have children by choice, and an 'i' shows infertility.

CHAPTER 6

NURSES' ROLE IN SCREENING, DIAGNOSIS AND FOLLOW UP

Due to a lack of awareness of FH by nurses and others in the healthcare industry worldwide, FH remains under-diagnosed and under-treated.

There have been numerous publications to date on the specific roles that clinical specialist nurses and nurse practitioner can play as a member of a collaborative healthcare team, both in primary care and within specialist clinics.

For example in 2008 the United Kingdom (UK) Department of Health established an FH cascade screening clinic following the positive conclusions of the 'Familial Hypercholestrolaemia Cascade Screening Research Study'.

The clinic is run by a 'Cascade Nurse Specialist' and caters for both adult and paediatric patients. Along with reduced clinic wait times it allows the nurse to follow up on lifestyle and risk factor management and to conduct cascade screening of family members at risk.

The successful establishment of this clinic in the UK is an excellent example of how specially trained nurses can play a pivotal role however, the authors believe all registered nurses can play a part in the identification and screening of FH patients without stepping outside their scope of practice.

In 2020 there was a FH Global Call to Action[31] to implement strategies to strive to close the gaps in identification and care of this common cause of preventable premature CVD and death. This publication highlighted 9 areas of priority that require action.

- Improve **Awareness** of FH in educational institutions, the medical community, the healthcare delivery system, and the general public.
- Improve **Advocacy** between partnerships of patients, physicians, and other healthcare professionals.
- Improve processes for **Screening, testing, and diagnosis** according to country-specific conditions and guidelines.
- Make **Treatment** for FH, made more available, affordable, and patient-centered.
- Develop **Separate guidelines for severe and homozygous FH**.

- Facilitate **Family-based care** with opportunities for greater patient involvement and shared decision-making.
- Develop more **Registries for research** into FH in order to qualify current practices and identify gaps between guidelines and healthcare delivery.
- Increase the level of scientific, genetic, epidemiologic, and clinical **Research** to improve FH care.
- Improve the **Cost and value** for families and societies, including improved quality of life.

All nurses working in primary care or in cardiac care areas of hospitals can play an important role in helping to facilitate attainment of many of these priorities by improving awareness of FH, patient advocacy, screening and identification of individuals who are at risk, and educating patients on lifestyle changes and medication adherence.

CHAPTER 7

RATIONALE FOR TREATMENT

Reducing the LDL-C level, which plays a causal role in the initiation and development of ASCVD, is one of the main goal of treatments. Therefore, in conjunction with lifestyle changes, maximally tolerated statin therapy, which is the mainstay for treatment of elevated cholesterol, should be started as early as possible.

Treatment Options

- Lifestyle changes:
    - Diet should be low in saturated fats. Low carbo-hydrate and keto-genic diets should be avoided.
    - exercise and NO smoking
- Drugs: Statins, Ezetimibe, Resins
- Nutraceuticals (e.g., red yeast)
- PCSK9 inhibitors

- LDL apheresis (used in severe HeFH, HoFH and high Lp(a) with progressive CAD)
- Novel therapies (e.g., Inclisiran which is approved for use in Australia. Evinacumab and Lomitapide are available through the TGA's special access scheme).

Statin Therapy

In all adult patient with FH, treatment options should initially aim to reduce the LDL-C level by 50%[27, 32, 33]. The statins available in Australia are listed below together with the daily dose ranges.

Low to Moderate intensity	**Daily dose lowers LDL-C by 30 – 50%**
Pravastatin (Pravachol)	20–40 mg (starting dose in adults) *(Approved for children>10yrs, starting dose 20mg)*
Atorvastatin (Lipitor)	10–40 mg (starting dose in adults) *(Approved for children>10yrs, starting dose 10mg)*
Simvastatin (Zocor)	5–40 mg (starting dose in adults)
Rosuvastatin (Crestor)	5–20 mg (starting dose in adults)

After reaching the 50% reduction target the following therapeutic goals for both HeFH and HoFH should be considered according to a patient's level of ASCVD risk:

1. LDL-C<2.5 mmol/L (absence of ASCVD or other major ASCVD risk factors);
2. LDL-C<1.8 mmol/L (imaging evidence of ASCVD alone or other major ASCVD risk factors); or
3. LDL-C<1.4 mmol/L (presence of clinical ASCVD)

High intensity	Daily dose lowers LDL-C by ≥ 50%
Atorvastatin	40–80 mg
Rosuvastatin	20–40 mg

In FH patients who develop a recurrent ASCVD event within 2 years on maximally tolerated statins, a lower primary target for LDL-C of <1.0 mmol/L may be considered[35].

Lifestyle changes

It is imperative that lifestyle modification is addressed for a minimum of 3 months for newly diagnosed HeFH patients and then a repeat full fasting cholesterol blood profile should be undertaken prior to commencing medication therapy. However, this does not apply for HeFH patients who have already suffered a ACS, MI or PCI or for those with HoFH.

Other Drug Therapies

If target LDL-C is not reached on statin therapy alone, which will often be the case in FH, then ezetimibe (e.g., Ezetrol) therapy is indicated.

If a patient is statin intolerant or resistant to using a statins then ezetimibe can be used alone or in combination with low dose intermittent statin dosing. In specialist centres other therapies may be considered.

PCSK9 Inhibitor therapy (evolocumab, alirocumab)

Proprotein convertase subtilisin/kexin type 9 (PCSK9)[14], is a protein that attaches to the LDL receptor and blocks the intracellular regeneration of the LDL receptor that is bound to LDL, which results in a reduction of LDC receptor numbers. So, blocking this action with PCSK9 inhibitors allows more receptors to be available on the surface of the liver cell resulting in a lowering of LDL-C in the blood. These therapies are administered as a subcutaneous injection either fortnightly or monthly.

Patients with diagnosed FH must meet specific criteria to be able to gain access to PCSK9 injections via the Pharmaceutical Benefits Scheme (PBS) and it must be prescribed by or in conjunction with a specialist.

Inclisiran (Leqvio | Therapeutic Goods Administration)

Inclisiran (Leqvio) is a new class of medicine known as a 'gene silencing' drug. It boosts the liver's ability to remove harmful cholesterol from the blood by turning off or 'silencing' the gene PCSK9. The Australian TGA has given provisional approval for this drug to be used in HeFH patients who have CVD or who are at high risk of a cardiovascular event. Inclisiran is expected to be listed on the Australian PBS in 2024. This therapy is administered as a subcutaneous injection initially, repeated at three months and then at six monthly intervals.

Evolving Models of Care and Treatment

The body of knowledge about FH has grown exponentially over the past decade since earlier models of care on screening, detection, diagnosis, treatment and management of FH patients where published[27, 36].

In order for this knowledge to continue to grow it requires further research, education and up-skilling of the health workforce in how to make an accurate and precise clinical diagnosis of FH[27, 33].

The most contemporary, international, evidence-based guidance for implementing best practice in the care of patients with FH was published in June 2023[36].

This guidance provides comprehensive recommendations for the best clinical care for people with FH worldwide, including treatment algorithms that should be considered for patients with HeFH and HoFH. The following two simplified diagrams (Figure 6 and 7) have been adapted from the guidelines[36].

Figure 6 Simplified treatment guide for patients with HeFH

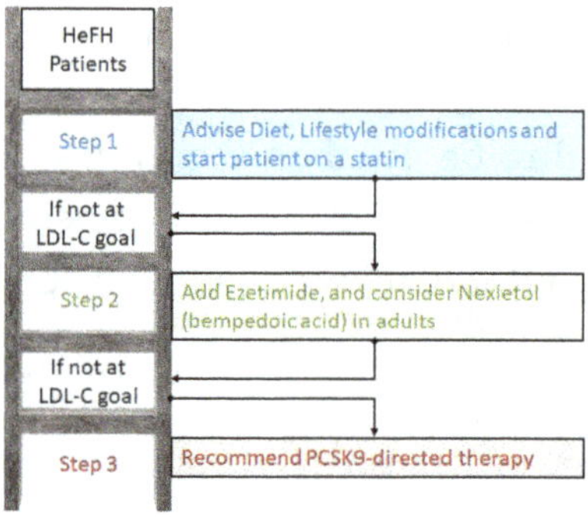

PCSK9 may be considered in children and adolescents with additional risk factors for atherosclerotic CVD, noting there is limited long term safety data[36].

Figure 7 Simplified treatment guide for patients with HoFH

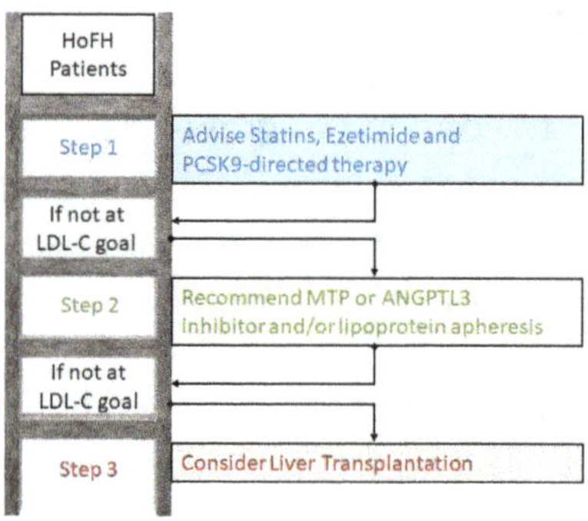

MTP and ANGPTL3 inhibitor are evolving modalities of treatment and there use in HoFH will be dependent on availability, preference, expertise and cost[36].

CHAPTER 8

INDEX CASE STUDY

A 30 year old, newly engaged, male with a family history of heart disease decided to have a cholesterol health check after a discussion with a colleague who also had elevated cholesterol levels. His initial fasting lipid profile results when first seen in 2018 were as follows:

Test	Results	Normal Ranges
Total Cholesterol (TC)	7.5 mmol/L	< 5.5 mmol/L
Triglycerides (Tg)	2.8 mmol/L	< 2.0 mmol/L
HDL	1.3 mmol/L	> 1.0 mmol/L
LDL-C	4.9 mmol/L	< 2.0 mmol/L
Lp(a)	216 nmol/L	< 72 nmol/L
ApoB	1.4 g/L	< 1.0 g/L

at initial consultation with a Nurse Practitioner

Height	167 cm
Weight	68 kg
BMI	24.4 kg/ m^2
Waist	84cm (central adiposity)
Country of Birth	Australia
Ethnicity	Mixed European and Chinese.
BP (right arm)	124 / 76
BP (left arm)	127 / 78
Smoking History	Never smoked
Diet	Asian cuisine predominately (not really heart healthy)
Alcohol	2 Alcohol Free Days a week; 2-3 beers on other days
Exercise	Exercise fanatic (gym, running, motor cycle and car racing)
Physical Examination	• No tendon Xanthomata • Bilateral Corneal Arcus from a young age • Heart sounds normal • Chest clear • Abdomen soft, non-tender/ BS present

He had no other personal medical history of relevance to a diagnosis of FH.

Family Medical History of Index Case

Mother

Of Singaporean Chinese ethnicity and was diagnosed with phenotypic FH in Singapore at a young age. Also had elevated cholesterol levels diagnosed in her early 50's and had a slightly elevated Lp(a) of 76nmol/L when tested. Mother's sister also diagnosed with FH, had AMI and stents aged 53.

Father

Of Welsh and Scottish ethnicity with no history of elevated cholesterol but did have an elevated Lp(a) level of 110nmol/L. He suffered an AMI and had stents inserted aged 48. Father's brother had elevated cholesterol levels diagnosed in his 50s.

Initial Therapeutic Treatment for Index Case

Rosuvastatin 5mg 3 times a week was commenced and then slowly titrated up to daily. Over time the dosage was increased to Rosuvastatin 10mg daily. He was also commenced on Ezetimibe 10mg which again was titrated up from 3 times a week to daily. Due to his family history of heart disease he was commenced on Aspirin 100mg daily.

This patient remained tolerant and compliant with his medications. Repeat Fasting Lipids tests in 2022 (after 4 years on treatment) were as follows and his Liver and Renal Function tests were within normal range.

Test	Results	Normal Ranges
Total Cholesterol (TC)	4.1 mmol/L	< 5.5 mmol/L
Triglycerides (Tg)	2.3 mmol/L	< 2.0 mmol/L
HDL	1.3 mmol/L	> 1.0 mmol/L
LDL-C	1.7 mmol/L	< 2.0 mmol/L

This patient's medications at the time of publication were Rosuvastatin 10mg daily, Ezetimibe 10mg daily, Aspirin 100mg daily. He continues to be followed up by a nurse practitioner every 6 months.

Cascade Screening of Family Members

The patient's father, mother, sister, one paternal aunt and one maternal aunt all agreed to have fasting Lipids, Lp(a) and ApoB tests performed. One paternal aunt and one maternal uncle refused testing.

The patient's 29 year old sister was found to have an LDL-C of 3.9mmol/L, Lp(a) of 87nmol/L, and an ApoB of 1.07. She has one child and is planning to have more so has opted not to commence therapeutic treatment at this time and is being managed by her GP. Both parents are also being managed by their GP.

The patient has a son who was born in 2021, 3 years after his initial diagnosis. He will have his son tested opportunistically if he requires blood testing or alternatively will have him tested around the age of 8 years.

Index Case Study Pedigree

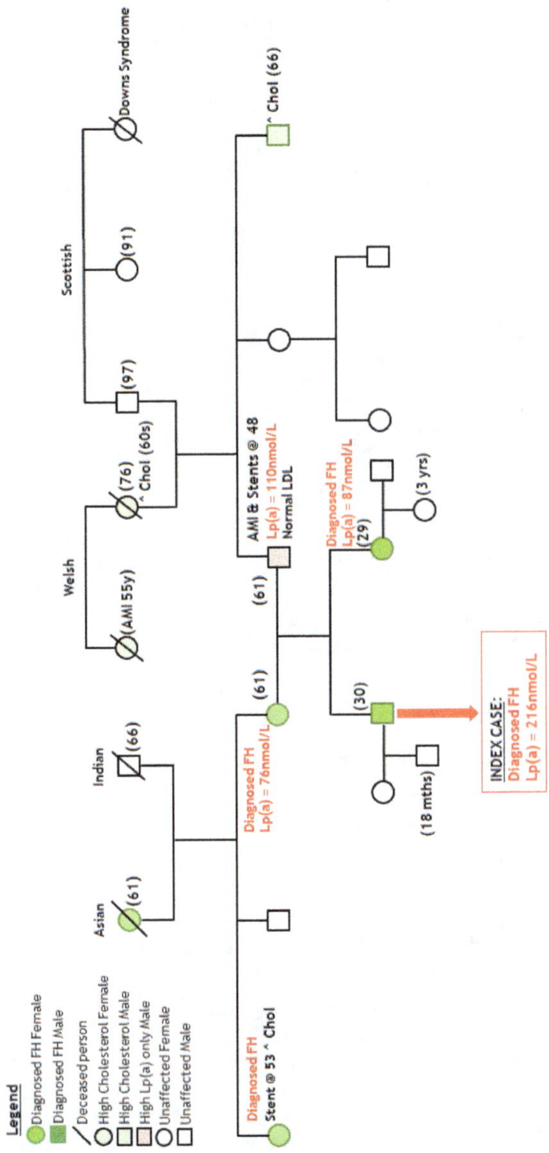

GLOSSARY OF TERMS

(Adapted from FH Australasia Network Website)

Angina
Pain or discomfort which occurs when the heart does not receive adequate blood flow. Angina may be experienced in the chest, neck, jaw, arms, shoulder or back.

Angiopoietin-related protein (ANGPTL3)
Is a liver derived circulating protein factor that inhibits the enzyme lipoprotein lipase. Researchers have been investigating antisense oligonucleotide and monoclonal antibody-based inactivation of ANGPTL3 in human clinical trials for the therapeutic management of dyslipidaemia and atherosclerosis[37].

Apolipoprotein
Protein component of lipoproteins.
Fat (lipo) + protein = lipoprotein

- **Apolipoprotein A1:** major protein component of HDL.
- **Apolipoprotein B:** protein component of LDL.

Atheroma

LDL cholesterol deposits in the wall of the arteries, also called plaque.

Atherosclerosis

The process where LDL cholesterol is deposited in the walls of the arteries causing them to narrow and eventually become blocked.

Autosomal dominant

Means you only need to get the 'faulty' gene from one parent in order for you to inherit the condition.

Bile acids

The liver produces bile acids from cholesterol. Bile acids are excreted into the intestine when we eat. Bile acids help fat to be absorbed.

Bile acid binding resins

A group of medications that lower cholesterol by working in the intestine.

BMI (Body Mass Index)

Is a quick way to check weight status e.g. to determine if you are a healthy weight for your height.

Cardiovascular

Relates to the heart (cardio) and blood vessels (vascular).

Cardiovascular disease

Any disease of the heart and blood vessels. Atherosclerosis and high blood pressure are the most common cardiovascular diseases.

Cascade screening

Is a mechanism for identifying people at risk for FH by a process of systematic family tracing.

Cholesterol

A waxy substance that circulates in the blood and plays a role in the formation of plaque.

Cholesterol absorption inhibitors

A group of medications that lower cholesterol by reducing its reabsorption in the intestine.

Compound heterozygous FH

- If you inherit two 'faulty' LDL receptor genes from both of your parents (both parents have FH), then none of the LDL receptors work.
- If the two 'faulty' LDL receptor genes are different types, it is called compound heterozygous FH. This is a very rare and very serious form of FH.

There are over a 1,000 different types of LDL receptor mutations.

Corneal arcus (also known as arcus cornealis)

Cholesterol deposits in the cornea of the eye.

Coronary arteries

These are the arteries on the surface of the heart that bring fresh blood, carrying oxygen and nutrients to the heart muscle.

Coronary artery disease (CAD)
A condition in which the arteries supplying the heart muscle become narrowed or blocked by LDL cholesterol and lack of oxygen causes tissue damage.

Enzyme
A protein which helps to speed up chemical reactions in your body.

Familial Hypercholesterolaemia (FH)
FH is an inherited disorder, which caused high LDL cholesterol from birth. This results in an increased risk of cardiovascular diseases, specifically coronary artery disease at an early age (men before the age of 55 and women before the age of 60).

Family history
The family structure and relationships within the family, including information about diseases in family members e.g., age relatives developed cardiovascular disease, had heart attacks, died etc.

Gene
A unit of hereditary which is transferred from parent to child and carries some characteristic to the child e.g. 'how to make an LDL receptor'.

Gene Variant
A 'fault' or mutation in the genetic material which is passed from parent to child.

Heart attack

When one of the arteries supplying the heart muscle with blood is partly or totally blocked and the muscle is not getting sufficient oxygen resulting in tissue damage.

Heterozygous FH

If you inherited one 'faulty' LDL receptor gene from one of your parents, 50% of your LDL receptors don't work.

High Density Lipoprotein (HDL)

Is the 'good' cholesterol because it helps to protect against cardiovascular disease.

Homozygous FH

If you inherit two 'faulty' LDL receptor genes from both of your parents (both parents have FH), then none of the LDL receptors work. If the two 'faulty' LDL receptor genes are the same type it is called homozygous FH. This is a very rare and very serious form of FH.

LDL receptor

The 'door' which allows the LDL cholesterol to be moved from the blood into the liver.

Lipids

Another name for fats.

Lipoprotein

A combination of fat and protein that transports lipids (fats) in the blood.

Lipoprotein (a) - pronounced as Lp little a
A genetic variation of LDL cholesterol. Lp(a) is not well understood but high levels are associated with increased risk of cardiovascular disease.

Lipoprotein apheresis
Is a treatment, similar to dialysis for renal patients, to reduce the LDL-C, and occasionally Lp(a), in the blood.

Low Density Lipoprotein (LDL)
Is called 'bad' cholesterol because it increases the risk of cardiovascular disease.

mmol/L
A unit of measurement, used in Australia to describe how much of a substance is in the blood e.g. LDL-C is 2.5mmol/L.

Microsomal triglyceride transfer protein (MTP)
Is required for the production of apoB containing lipoproteins by the liver and the intestine. It is responsible for the hepatic assembly of VLDL particles through the transfer of triglycerides to apolipoprotein B. Genetic variants in MTP result in a rare genetic disorder called Abetalipoproteinemia, which leads to malabsorption and severe deficiencies in the fat soluble vitamins (A, D, E and K)[38].

Peripheral artery disease
A condition in which the arteries supplying the peripheral parts (not heart and brain) of the body become narrowed or blocked and lack of oxygen causes tissue damage e.g. leg

pain when walking (intermittent claudication) and erectile dysfunction in men.

Plant sterols

Sterols and cholesterol are similar in structure, so they compete for absorption in the small intestine; the plant sterols stop the cholesterol from being absorbed.

Plaque

Are deposits of cholesterol in the walls of the arteries. The plaque builds up and narrows the artery.

Predictive genetic testing

Refers to testing of an individual who currently does not have symptoms or signs of a condition, but who might be at an increased risk due to their family history.

Risk factor

Those factors which increase the likelihood of getting a disease. There are modifiable risk factors which can be changed by lifestyle and/or medication and non-modifiable risk factors which cannot be changed by lifestyle or medication.

Premature CVD

Is any disease of the heart and blood vessels that occurs prior to the age threshold of <55 years in males and <65 years in females, as defined in multiple clinical guidelines such as those published by the American College of Cardiology(ACC), the American Heart Association (AHA) and the European Society of Cardiology (ESC).

Statins
A group of medications that lower cholesterol by blocking its production in the liver.

Triglycerides
A type of fat found in the blood. High levels are associated with increased risk of cardiovascular disease.

Total cholesterol
The total amount of cholesterol in the blood; includes LDL, triglyceride and HDL.

Xanthomas
Cholesterol deposits commonly found in the tendons of the hand and the Achilles tendon and is often associated with high cholesterol levels.

Xanthomatosis
Is a condition in which fatty deposits occur in various parts of the body.

REFERENCES

1. Muller C. Xanthomata, hypercholesterolemia, angina pectoris. *Acta Med Scand*. 95 1938; 89: 75– 84
2. Khachadurian AK. 1964 The inheritance of essential familial hypercholestrolemia. *Am J Med.* 137: 402-407.
3. Khachadurian AK, Uthman SM. 1973 Experiences with the homozygous case of familial hypercholestrolemia. A Report of 52 patients. *Nutr Metab.* 15. 132-140.
4. Goldstein JL, Brown MS. Familial hypercholesterolemia: identification of a defect in the regulation of 3-hydroxy-3-methylglutaryl coenzyme A reductase activity associated with overproduction of cholesterol. *Proc Natl AcadSci USA.* 1973; *70*: 2804–2808
5. Brown MS, Goldstein JL. Familial hypercholesterolemia: defective binding of lipoproteins to cultured fibroblasts associated with impaired regulation of 3-hydroxy-3- methylglutaryl coenzyme A reductase activity. *Proc Natl AcadSci USA.* 1974; *71*: 788–792

6. Goldstein JL, Brown MS. The low-density lipoprotein pathway and its relation to atherosclerosis. *Ann RevBiochem.*1977;*46*: 897–930
7. Brown MS, Goldstein JL. Receptor-mediated endocytosis: Insights from lipoprotein receptor system. *Proc Natl AcadSci USA.* 1979; 76: 3330-3337
8. Brown MS, Goldstein JL. How LDL receptors influence cholesterol and atherosclerosis. *Sci Am.* 1984; *251*: 58–66
9. Ose L. The Real Code of Leonardo da Vinci. *CurrCardiol Rev.* 2008 Feb; 4(1): 60-62
10. Goldstein JL, Brown MS. The LDL Receptor *Atheroscler Thromb Vasc Bio.* 2009
11. Austin MA, Hutter CM, Zimmern RL, Humphries SE. Genetic causes of monogenic heterozygous familial hypercholesterolemia: a HuGE prevalence review. *Am J Epidemiol.* 2004 Sep 1;160 (5):407-20.
12. Matthews L. Variation in the Prevalence of Familial Hypercholestrolemia Around the World. *J Am Coll Cardio.* 2015 Jul: 17.08.
13. De Castro-Orós I, Pocoví M, Civeira F. The genetic basis of familial hypercholesterolemia: inheritance, linkage, and mutations. *ApplClin Genet.* 2010 Aug 5;3:53-64
14. Horton JD, Cohen JC, Hobbs HH. PCSK9: a convertase that coordinates LDL catabolism. *J Lipid Res.* 2009 Apr; 50 (Suppl): S172-S177

15. Beheshti SO, Madsen CM, Varbo A et.al. Worldwide Prevalence of Familial Hypercholesterolemia. Meta-Analyses of 11 Million Subjects. *J Am Coll Cardiol.* 2020; 75:2553-66.

16. Henderson R, O'Kane M, McGilligan V, Watterson S. The genetics and screening of familial hypercholesterolaemia. *J Biomed Sci.* 2016; 23: 39.

17. Pang J, Chan DC, Hu M, Muir LA, et.al. Comparative aspects of the care of familial hypercholesterolemia in the "Ten Countries Study" *J. Clin. Lipid.* (2019) 13, 287-300.

18. Chen P, Chen X and Zhang S. Current Status of Familial Hypercholesterolemia in China: A Need for Patient FH Registry Systems. *Front. Physiol.* 2019 10:280

19. Horton AE, Martin AC, Srinivasan S, et al. Integrated guidance to enhance the care of children and adolescence with Familial Hypercholestrolaemia: Practical advice for the community clinician. *J Paediatric & Child Health.* 58 (2022) 1297-1312

20. Sijbrands EJG, Westendorp RGJ, Defesche JC, et al. Mortality over two centuries in a large pedigree with familial hypercholesterolaemia: family tree mortality study. *Heart Lung Circ.* April 2001, Vol322; 1019-1023

21. Wiegman A, Gidding SS, et al. Familial hypercholesterolaemia in children and adolescents: gaining decades of life by optimizing detection and treatment. *Eur Heart J.* 2015; 36: 2425-2437

22. Schmidt EB, Hedegaard BS, Retterstol K. Familial hypercholestrolaemia: history, diagnosis, screening, management and challenges. *Heart.* 2020 Dec:106(24): 1940-46

23. Nordestgaard BG, Chapman MJ, Humphries SE, et al. Familial hypercholesterolaemia is underdiagnosed and undertreated in the general population: guidance for clinicians to prevent coronary heart disease: consensus statement of the European Atherosclerosis Society. *Eur Heart J.* 2013; 34. 3478–90a.

24. Yuan G, Wang J, et al. Heterozygous familial hypercholesterolemia: an underrecognized cause of early cardiovascular disease. *CMAJ.* 2006 174-178

25. Borén J, Chapman MJ, Krauss RM, et.al. Low-density lipoproteins cause atherosclerotic cardiovascular disease: pathophysiological, genetic, and therapeutic insights: a consensus statement from the European Atherosclerosis Society Consensus Panel. *Eur. Heart J.* 2020 41, 2313–2330

26. Cuchel M, Bruckert E, Ginsberg HN, et al. Homozygous familial hypercholesterolaemia: new insights and guidance for clinicians to improve detection and clinical management. A position paper from the Consensus Panel on Familial Hypercholesterolaemia of the European Atherosclerosis Society. *Eur Heart J.* 2014; 35: 2146-2157.

27. Watts GF, Sullivan DR, Poplawski N, et al. Familial hypercholesterolaemia: A model of care for Australasia. *Atheroscler. Suppl.* 2011; 12(2): 221–63.

28. Watts GF. Gidding S, Wierzbicki AS, et al. Integrated guidance on the care of familial hypercholesterolaemia from the International FH Foundation. Int. *J. Cardiol.* 171, 309–325 (2014).

29. Brett T, Arnold-Reed D. Familial hypercholesterolaemia: A guide for general practice. *AJGP.* Sep 2019 Vol. 48, No. 9, 650-652.

30. Ellis KL, Pang J, Shultz CJ, Watts GF. New data on familial hypercholesterolaemia and acute coronary syndromes: The promise of PCSK9 monoclonal antibodies in the light of recent clinical trials. *EJPC.* 2017, Vol. 24(11) 1200–1205.

31. Representatives of the Global Familial Hypercholesterolemia Community; Wilemon KA, Patel J, Aguilar-Salinas C, Ahmed CD et.al. Reducing the Clinical and Public Health Burden of Familial Hypercholesterolemia: A Global Call to Action. *JAMA Cardiol.* 2020 Feb 1;5 (2):217-229.

32. Watt GF, Sullivan DR, Hare DL, et.al. Integrated Guidance for Enhancing the Care of Familial Hypercholesterolaemia in Australia. *Heart Lung Circ.* (2021) 30, 324–349.

33. Cesaro A, Fimiani F, Gragnano F, et al., New Frontiers in the treatment of Homozygous Familial

Hypercholestrolemia. *Heart Failure Clin.* 2022 Jan: 18(1): 18.177-188

34. Watts GF, Gidding SS, Hegele RA, et al. International Atherosclerosis Society guidance for implementing best practice in the care of familial hypercholesterolaemia. *Nat Rev Cardiol.* (2023) https://doi.org/10.1038/s41569-023-00892-0.

35. Pang J, Lansberg PJ, Watts GF. International Developments in the Care of Familial Hypercholesterolaemia: Where Now and Where to Next? *J Atheroscler Thromb.* 2016; 23: 505-519

36. Watts GF, Gidding SS, Matta P, Pang J. et al. Familial Hypercholestrolaemia: evolving knowledge for designing adaptive models of care. *Nat Rev Cardiol.* 17, 360–377 (2020).

37. Kersten S. Angiopoietin-like 3 in lipoprotein metabolism. *Nat Rev Endocrinol.* 13, 731–739 (2017).

38. Wang J, Hegele RA, Microsomal triaglyceride transfer protein (MTP) gene mutations in Canadian subjects with abetalipoproteinemia. *Hum. Mutat.* (2000) 15 (3): 294–5.

USEFUL LINKS

FH Australasia Network

https://www.athero.org.au/fh

The FH Australasia Network's mission is to prevent early heart attacks in people with inherited high cholesterol by means of:

- identification, diagnosis and treatment of genetic cholesterol disorders for patients and their affected relatives
- educating patients, health care providers and government agencies and fostering patient support
- encouraging research to increase understanding and treatment of genetic cholesterol disorders
- promoting public health efforts fostering collaboration between agencies and other health care providers.

FH Health Professionals and Specialists

https://www.athero.org.au/fh/health-professionals/fh-specialists

A list of health professional that specialise in the diagnosis, management and treatment of patients with lipid disorders and FH.

FH Europe

https://fheurope.org/

Is the leading European charity that focuses on patient advocacy and has a wealth of resources.

Heart Foundation

http://heartfoundation.org.au/

Is the leading Australian charity that provides a wealth of resources for health professionals and the community on all aspects of cardiovascular disease.

Heart Support-Australia

http://heartnet.org.au/

This organisation helps Australians to maintain strong hearts through peer support, information and encouragement. Heart Support-Australia help people affected by heart conditions achieve excellent health outcomes.

Heart UK

http://heartuk.org.uk/

Is the leading UK cholesterol charity that provides extensive resources for health professionals, patients and families on all aspects of the detection and management of FH. They also provide undergraduate and postgraduate courses for health professionals online for those living outside of the UK.

National Lipid Association (NLA) USA

http://www.lipid.org/

Is a US based multidisciplinary specialty society providing education on detection and management of dyslipidaemia and related disorders.

Learn Your Lipids

http://www.learnyourlipids.com/

This site provides information for patients with dyslipidaemia which includes those with FH.

British Heart Foundation

http://www.bhf.org.uk/

Is a leading British foundation that provides excellent resources for health professionals and patients, including informative videos on a wide spectrum of conditions and risk factors.

NSW Genetic Service

http://www.genetic.edu.au/

The educational arm of NSW Genetic Service provides genetic information for individuals and their families affected by genetic conditions and health professionals who work with them.

Nurse Managed Lipid Clinics video

https://nursemanagedlipidclinics.com/

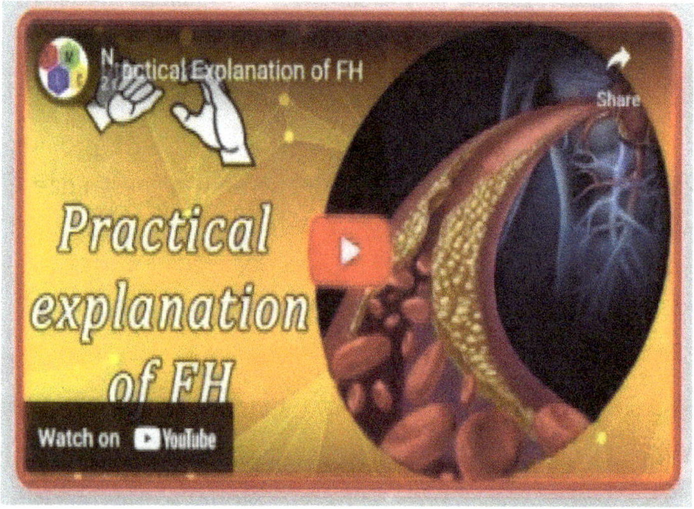

ENDORSEMENTS

"I have been working in CCU now for a few years and after being invited to review it, I feel 'A Pocket Guide of FH for Nurses' would be highly beneficial to access when educating patients and clinical staff. I found it very easy to read and it gives all essential and relevant information needed to understand FH. I liked the historical journey covering the genetics of FH, its' diagnosis, management and treatments.

The Guide's colour images make it easier to visually identify the signs and symptoms. I feel this Guide will be an essential resource for RNs and RMOs in the CCU setting. The tools provided in the Guide are designed to be utilised on a daily basis to help clinicians to be confident in looking out for patients with undiagnosed FH."

Judy Tito
Clinical Nurse ICU/CCU

"A Pocket Guide of FH for Nurses is a great resource for nurses and clinicians alike in understanding, identifying and in the management of FH. I found chapters 3 and 4 extremely useful covering the essentials clearly and concisely. I will certainly refer to it now in my practice"

Anu Joyson, RN, MN, NP student
Hypertension Specialist Centre

ACKNOWLEDGEMENTS

Every author needs a reason to get started. For us the idea of this pocket guide was first mooted during the three years we worked together at the UWA's School of Medicine and Pharmacology based at Royal Perth Hospital.

The authors wish to sincerely thank Prof. Gerald Watts and Prof. Frank Van Bockxmeer for improving our clinical knowledge and understanding of lipid disorders, and in particular the genetically inherited disorder FH.

Having learned so much about FH, it was the desire to continue to inform, educate, empower, and encourage our nursing colleagues to play a pivotal role in identifying those individuals, who are at higher risk of early onset coronary artery disease due to FH, that was the impetus for writing this book.

The authors wish to sincerely thank Dr. Warrick Bishop, for his continued encouragement and support during the development and publication of this book.

To our colleagues, Judith Bruechert, Judy Tito, and Anu Joyson our grateful thanks for their review and valuable feedback of the first drafts.

www.ingramcontent.com/pod-product-compliance
Lightning Source LLC
La Vergne TN
LVHW020325220926
848484LV00001BB/1
* 9 7 8 0 6 4 8 6 2 7 0 5 0 *